Nobody's Home

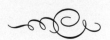

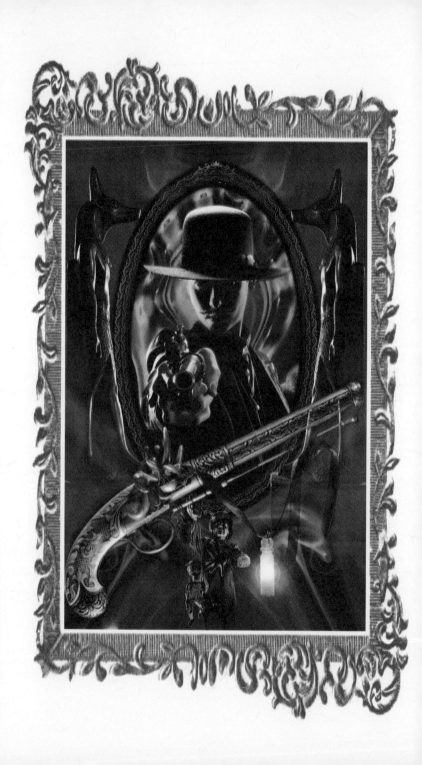

Nobody's Home:

An Anubis Gates Story

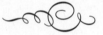

Tim Powers

Illustrated by J. K. Potter

Subterranean Press 2014

First Edition

Trade Edition ISBN
978-1-59606-670-0

Limited Edition ISBN
978-1-59606-671-7

Subterranean Press
PO Box 190106
Burton, MI 48519

subterraneanpress.com

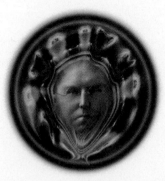

"Eternal process moving on,
From state to state the spirit walks;
And these are but the shattered stalks,
Or ruined chrysalis of one."

—Tennyson, *In Memoriam*

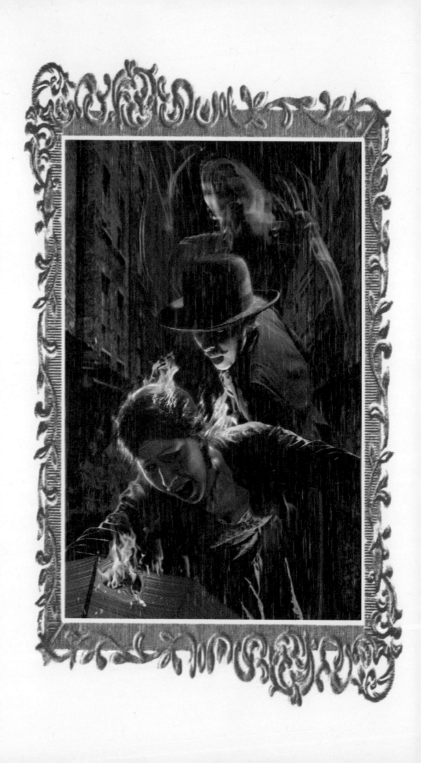

OVER THE CLATTER of rain on the canvas awning above her head and the more remote background hiss of it on the pavement of Cannon Street in the darkness below, she could hear a faint, repeated crunching splash, as if someone were laboriously plodding down the narrow, gravel-paved street; but the sound didn't change its position.

Jacky Snapp shifted forward on the stone ledge and peered down. A streetlamp raised yellow gleams on an umbrella a dozen feet below her and to her left, out in front of St. Swithin's Church, and the umbrella was bouncing up and down as it moved forward eight steps, then stopped, whirled and jumped eight steps back.

Midnight was long past, and the London streets were quiet except for the occasional rattle of a carriage and horses, or a distant bell from out on the river. Jacky had spent the evening tracking down a beggar who was rumored to have fur growing all over him like an ape, but when she had cornered the man in the basement of an old pub off Fleet Street, her hand tense on the flintlock pistol under her coat, he had turned out to be only a very hairy old fellow with a prodigious beard—not the half-legendary man she had devoted her life to finding and killing.

Another false trail.

Her cold hand went to her chest, and under the fabric of her shirt she felt the glass cylinder she wore on a ribbon around her neck. I won't give up, Colin, she thought—I promise.

The umbrella below her was still hopping back and forth on its eight-step course, and

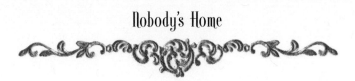
it occurred to her that the person holding it might be playing hopscotch, jumping through the pattern of squares in the children's game. Alone, at midnight, in the rain. Jacky had only arrived in the city a couple of weeks ago, but she was sure this must be uncommon.

She pushed her wide-brimmed hat more firmly down onto her cut-short hair and prodded the false moustache glued to her upper lip, then leaned out from the first-floor window ledge to grip the wet drain-pipe by which she had climbed up to this perch; it still felt solidly moored, so she swung out and slid down the cold metal till her boots stopped at a bracket. From here she could stretch a loose-trousered leg sideways onto the granite sill of a ground-floor window, and a moment later she had dropped lightly to the street.

The figure under the umbrella was a girl, facing away now, her wet skirt flapping around her ankles under the hem of a dark coat as she hopped forward on one foot.

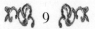

Jacky had decided simply to steal away in the other direction, toward the dim silhouette of St. Paul's cathedral dome, when the umbrella abruptly began to glow; in the same moment it was tossed aside and Jacky saw that bright flames had sprung up on the girl's shoulders and in her hair.

Jacky leaped forward and drove her shoulder into the girl's back, and when the girl tumbled forward onto her hands and knees on the wet gravel, Jacky pushed her over sideways and leaned in over the burning coat and tried to roll the girl's head into a puddle. The heat on Jacky's face made her squint and hold her breath, and her hands and wrists were scorching, and the glass vial had fallen out of her shirt and was swinging in the flames.

And another person was crouched beside her, trying to push her hands back; Jacky swung a fist in the person's direction, but it connected with nothing but cold rainy air. Finally she was able to roll the girl over onto her back,

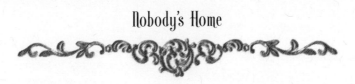
extinguishing the coat, and with stinging hands splash water onto the girl's head.

With the flames put out, the street seemed darker than ever; Jacky flinched to see glowing spots on the pavement, but at a second glance she saw that they only shone a dim green. Even as she blinked at them they faded, but not before she noticed that they had been arranged in a long row of foot-wide rectangles.

Hopscotch! she thought. She leaned back, gasping in the wonderfully cold air, and quickly looked around, but whoever it was who had tried to interfere in her rescue was gone. The girl lying on the street was panting and moving feebly.

On its now-charred ribbon, the vial that hung around Jacky's neck was too hot to touch, so she let it swing free for now. She started to get to her feet—

And with a start she noticed figures standing in the dimness of an alley on the south side of the street, scarcely a dozen feet away from where she crouched. She couldn't tell how many.

They wavered in the rainy breeze, as if they were silhouettes painted on an unmoored canvas, but their hands were moving and their heads turned back and forth, perhaps in whispered conversation.

Jacky's face suddenly felt colder than the rain, and her ribs tingled. As cautiously as if the alley figures were a pack of feral dogs, Jacky took hold of the girl's still-hot lapels and pulled her to her feet.

"He was supposed to go," the girl was saying, but Jacky put one hand over her mouth and gripped her elbow with the other.

"Walk quiet," she whispered, and took a tense step away, toward St. Paul's.

But with a flutter like birds the shadowy silhouettes came spinning out of the alley. They seemed to suffer in the rain, squeaking and ducking and cringing, but Jacky yanked her companion around and shoved her toward the drain pipe and yelled, "Climb!"

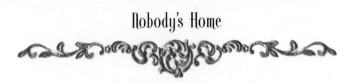

To her relief, the girl scrambled rapidly up the pipe, bracing her feet in the gaps between the blocks of the wall, and Jacky followed so closely that her head was between the girl's ankles until they had both scrambled onto the window ledge under the awning.

For several seconds neither of them spoke as they caught their breath.

Then, "You knew not to just run," panted the girl. "Away down the street."

Jacky was hugging herself and shivering. One of the things down there had been in profile for a moment, and the shape of the face, and the angle of the elbow and shoulder below it, had jarred her.

She touched the glass vial that dangled on her chest, and it was still too hot to tuck into her shirt.

The girl was sitting to her right, a foot away on the three-foot-wide ledge. "I should have let you burn," said Jacky bleakly as she flexed her stinging hands.

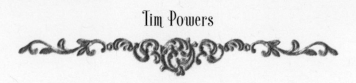

She looked down—the shadowy crowd was milling aimlessly on the narrow street between St. Swithin's on one side and a dark chemist's shop on the other. She looked away quickly.

The girl pulled her knees up and clasped her arms around them. "Can we get up to the roof from here?"

"Why? Those are...*ghosts*, aren't they? Whatever *you* are, catching fire in the street like that." Jacky was trying to fit into her experience the idea that she had apparently actually seen ghosts, and even perhaps one particular ghost, and she hoped she wasn't going to giggle or start crying. "Ghosts can only see footprints, I've heard," she went on, remembering the girl's earlier remark. "That's why I didn't run."

The girl nodded. "My name's Harriet. Living folk will be drawn to this, and living folk are likely to look up." She turned toward Jacky, and even in the deep shadow Jacky could see Harriet's wide eyes and pinched

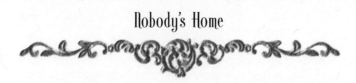
mouth. "And it's not a kindly sort of living folks who'd be drawn to it."

Jacky took a deep breath and exhaled, then nodded and touched her false moustache to make sure it was secure against more rain. "I'm Jacky," she said. Then she got up on her knees and leaned out to grip the drain-pipe again. "On up the pipe for two more floors. Don't slip."

She led the way this time, pushing herself upward with the edges of her boots between the blocks and letting the cold wet pipe slide soothingly through her linked hands and trying to peer upward through the rain, and after two welcomely distracting minutes of the strenuous exercise she had swung a leg over the cornice and rolled across the coping and landed on all fours on a tar-papered roof.

A moment later Harriet landed on top of her.

Jacky pushed her off and then leaned back against the low wall, scowling. The night was not as dark up here above the

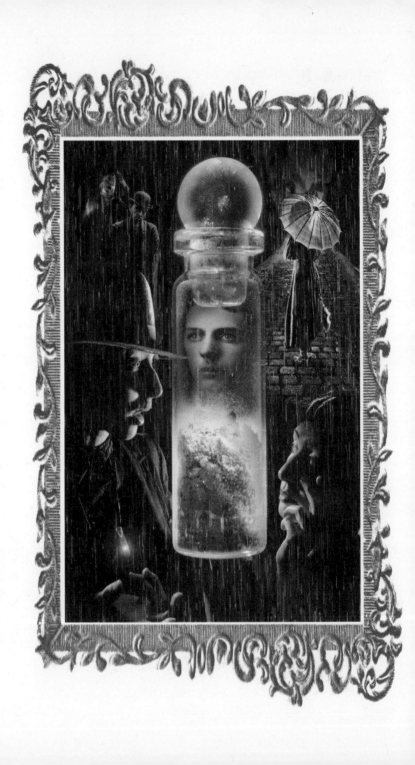

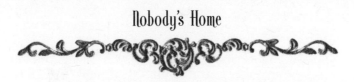
street, and she could see that Harriet was not much older than herself—perhaps nineteen or twenty.

Jacky dug a pewter flask out from an inside pocket of her coat—the back of her hand brushed the glass vial, which was still hot—and unscrewed the cap gingerly with her burned fingers.

After she had taken a long swallow of the warm brandy, she passed the flask to her companion, who was now sitting cross-legged a yard away. The rain was abating, and a less-dark patch in the clouds overhead might have been the emerging moon.

Harriet tilted the flask up and took a long sip. "You saved me from burning to death," she said hoarsely, exhaling. "Thank you."

Jacky shrugged. "I don't think you'd have burned to *death*," she said, "with the rain and all." She wagged her hand for the flask, and Harriet passed it back to her.

"Oh he'd have made sure of it," said Harriet with a visible shudder. "My husband's

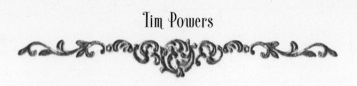

ghost—he even tried to push you off me when you were trying to put me out." She shook her head, her wet hair flapping around her narrow face. Perhaps talking to herself more than to Jacky, she went on softly, "I don't know what I'm going to *do!* That hopscotch in front of the London Stone was supposed to send him off to Purgatory. Or Hell."

Jacky recalled that a round piece of rock called the London Stone, about the size of a watermelon, was mounted in an alcove beside the front doors of St. Swithin's Church. "Why did—" she began.

But Harriet had been peering at Jacky's face, and now interrupted her. "Why've you got a sham moustache on?"

Jacky felt as if her life were unravelling tonight. The wrong hairy man at the pub, the disturbing ghost in the street, and now her necessary disguise seemed to be useless.

"Sham?" she said, belatedly remembering to speak in her usual assumed lower pitch.

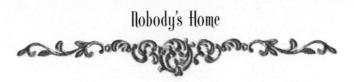

"And the short hair." Harriet touched a bristly patch on her own scalp. "Though I'm one to talk, now."

"Er...I don't know what you—"

"Go on, I watched how you moved when you were climbing," Harriet said. "And your voice, till just now. You're a girl. Why the fakery?"

"Oh, hell." Jacky sighed and abandoned the pretense. "I, uh, have to mingle with some rough folk, in bad places. A girl would be...at a disadvantage."

"Have to?"

Jacky took another mouthful of brandy from the flask instead of answering. Then she bust out, "What—*happened*, down there?"

"Your waked-up ghost got tangled with mine," said Harriet, "my husband, when you knocked me down. And that pretty much got a whole lot of 'em waked up."

"My waked-up ghost?" Colin, she thought, does she mean *you?* Don't have been that ghost in the street, please! Stay—remote.

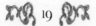

"Somebody whose ghost you're tied to," said Harriet. "Husband?"

"I'm not married!"

"Well, common-law, or any sort of, you know, informal but consummated. Your body is where you...*overlapped* with him."

"I—we—never did. That. We were engaged to be married. He was a poet," she added.

"Oh. Somebody else then?"

Jacky shook her head.

"You're a virgin? Then you must be carrying around a piece of him...?" She stared at Jacky curiously.

"No! Wait—" She touched the glass vial, which was impossibly still hot. "I—took his—dottle."

Harriet's eyes were wide. "You took his *head?*"

Jacky couldn't help barking out one syllable of a laugh. "Not noddle, *dottle*. The ash from a clay pipe of his." She pointed at the glass vial. "Ceneromancy, it's called. Magic

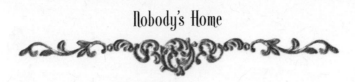
you do with ashes. It's kept him near me, since…since he was killed."

Near enough for me to feel his presence, at least, she thought, and for him to put up lines of his poetry into my head when I'm nearly asleep—but not to appear in front of me, *looking* at me!

Harriet reached out hesitantly, and when Jacky warned her that it was somehow still hot from having swung over the fire, she only brushed the vial with the back of a finger.

"Well that's how come your man's ghost got awake," she said, leaning back. "That fire on me was lit by my mad dead husband. He was a lascar from Dumdum in India, a sailor. We were married two-and-some years ago— Spring of 1807—and he couldn't go back to India because marrying me broke his caste, and he'd be killed for it. He was a decent enough husband, though our two babies were born dead, but after he died he turned horrid—he wants me to do sattee, do you know what that is?"

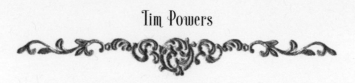
Jacky thought it might be some sort of curried Indian stew, but she shook her head.

"That's where they burn the widow of a dead man. He'd never have wanted such a thing when he was alive, and I think it's really for higher castes than what he was—but his damned ghost thinks he's a brahmin or something now, and fancies a proper escort to his, his *heathen hereafter*." She looked anxiously toward the edge of the roof as if she expected to see her husband's ghost come clambering over the cornice. The only sounds from the street, though, were faint echoes of someone running, clearly not a ghost.

Jacky handed her the flask, and when Harriet had finished it and handed it back empty, and Jacky had opened her coat to tuck it back into the inner pocket, Harriet sat back suddenly.

"You've got a gun?" she said.

"Oh. Well, yes." Jacky buttoned her coat self-consciously. "Like I said, I have to

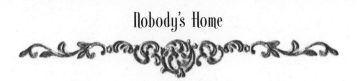
associate with some bad sorts sometimes." She stared at Harriet, then went on, speaking more rapidly, "I mean to find the man, the creature, that murdered Colin, my fiancee, and kill him. It's why I left home and came to London, it's why I can't be a girl while I'm here, looking for him in the low sort of places he's likely to be found. It's..." She rubbed her eyes, lowered her hands, and shrugged. "Well, to tell you the truth, it's all I've got left." She gave the other girl a frail smile. "Revenge."

"You know who he is, the man who murdered him?" Harriet seemed glad to be distracted from talk of her husband.

"Not in any...lasting sense."

"You know what he looks like?"

"Sometimes. But a description of him is only good for a couple of days. And sometimes he's covered with fur, like an ape."

Harriet's eyes were wide. "Are you joking?" When Jacky shook her head, Harriet went on, "You mean that werewolf, Doggy Joe? I thought he was made up."

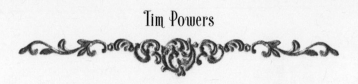
"Dog-Face Joe. And no, he's real enough. He's not a werewolf—he grows fur all over himself, because of some curse, but then he can switch bodies with you, so *you're* suddenly in his old furry body and he's in yours—" She paused to catch her breath, "—and just before he leaves his old body, he eats poison, so you—" Her voice faltered to a stop, and she looked away over the rooftop chimneys, blinking and biting her lip.

"And that's how your fellow died, this Colin?"

Jacky nodded.

"Well…damn. It's no use talking to his ghost, though. A ghost's just not the person it's a ghost of."

Jacky shuddered. "I don't want to talk to him. It."

Harriet seemed surprised by her vehemence.

Jacky stood up, a bit unsteadily. "Let's get down from here. There's bound to be an easier way at the back."

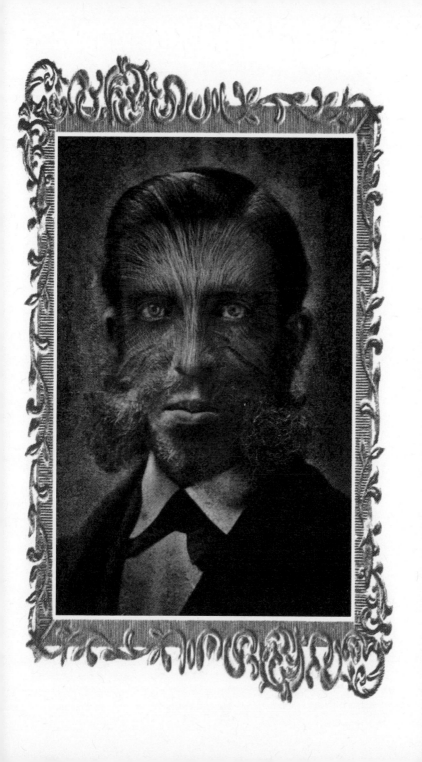

They descended one floor on an iron ladder bolted to the north side of the building, and then a fire escape with ornamental iron balusters led them to another ladder, which extended down to the pavement of a narrow alley. By the yellow glow in a couple of smoke-fogged windows they were able to pick their way over the wet cobblestones, around a right-angle turn, and then a silvery rectangle ahead showed them a moonlit segment of Cannon Street.

"I hope they're gone," whispered Jacky as they moved forward.

"Has your *dottle* cooled off?"

Jacky touched the pendant. "Maybe a bit. I *should* have let you burn."

Harriet exhaled shakily. "You might get another chance shortly."

But when they stepped out of the shadowed alley mouth onto the crushed gravel

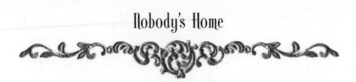

pavement of Cannon Street, it wasn't ghosts they met. Jacky saw a man sprint heavily past from right to left with a puppet jouncing on strings clutched in his fist, and then two men came loping along right behind him, their coats flapping. The men passed Jacky and Harriet standing in the alley mouth, but a moment later Jacky saw the jiggling puppet's head swivel around to face backward. Its little face was as sunken and folded as a dried apple, and moonlight glittered on a pair of spectacles attached over the withered nose.

One of the men behind apparently noticed the action, and his boots scraped on the gravel as he stopped and turned to look in the same direction.

"It's looking at those two," the man barked.

The one with the puppet looked toward Jacky and Harriet and nodded, then immediately sat down in the wet street and began crooning to the puppet and stroking its patchy scalp. The other two ran directly toward Jacky and her companion.

Jacky caught her balance and spun to run back down the dark alley, but a loud boom shook the air, and she looked back over her shoulder as the echoes batted away between the close building-fronts.

Her pursuers had halted, peering to Jacky's right, and an operatically deep voice from that direction called, "Not in Billingsgate, Thames Street or Cheapside, creepers!"

A prolonged metallic squeaking followed this, and Jacky caught Harriet's arm and whispered, "Hold up, I know this one."

The man with the puppet struggled to his feet. "You fired your gun," he said in a nasal voice. "And we're three and you got your legs off."

A low little wheeled cart rocked into view from the right, and on it sat a burly man with no legs, his face entirely hidden by a bushy dark beard and a big pair of spectacles and a cap pulled low over them. His massive arms

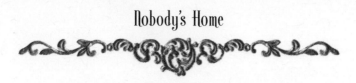

flexed as he braked by pressing his hands against the gravel.

"I've got another gun," he said; then he raised his hands and clenched them into big fists. "And I can break the legs off all three of you. Come and see if I can't."

The man stepped back and tucked his unsavory puppet under his coat. "Are you with Horrabin's beggars' guild or Captain Jack's?"

"Captain Jack's," said the legless man, "but one of Horrabin's lot probably sniffed this uproar too, and may shortly appear. Neither guild is happy with trespassing shade-dealers."

The three men darted venomous glances at Jacky and Harriet, but after a moment's hesitation they began walking away east on Cannon Street, and soon they were swaggering as if to show that they hadn't been intimidated.

The man on the cart wheeled around to face Jacky and Harriet. "And you two fools! Are you *trying* to get killed? You know how the shaders pluck awakened ghosts from haunted folk?"

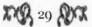

"Hullo, Skate," said Jacky, in her deeper voice.

The man pulled the spectacles off his face and peered. "Mother of God, young Jacky is it? When did you turn stupid? Parading around Eastcheap wearing a wide-awake ghost! Boy, you—"

"It wasn't wide-awake till this girl's dead husband tried to set her on fire!" protested Jacky. "Mine is ashes in a little flacon around my neck, and when I tried to *extinguish* her, it got heated up in *her* ghost's flames."

Skate hooked the spectacles on his nose again, then hastily took them off. "Yours is plenty lively now—it'll be kicking and blowing for days, I expect. And you," he said, squinting at Harriet, "why have you got your dead husband onstage?—especially if he wants to burn you up?"

"I was trying to hopscotch him off by the London Stone," said Harriet defensively.

"Ach, idiot child, that hasn't been a good trap-door since the stone broke in two in the

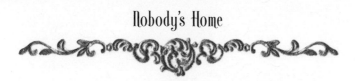
Great Fire—though it's still good enough to wake the lads up, worse luck." He shook his head. "Through the devil glasses you both shine like dishes of burning brandy. You can't walk the streets—the flash of you will draw more fellows like your man there with the mummied head on a puppet, and I *don't* actually have another gun." He snapped his fingers impatiently. "You don't dare leave footprints—even hopping on one foot's no good, as your friend found out." He sighed and shook his head.

Jacky touched the vial hanging outside her shirt, and it was still too hot to tuck in against her skin under the fabric. Kicking and blowing for *days?* she thought in alarm.

After a pause, Skate said, "There's no help for it. Have you got two shillings?"

"Yes," said Jacky. "They're rightfully the Captain's, though. I got 'em doing the thimble and pea trick in a pub."

"I'll acquaint Captain Jack with the circumstances," said Skate. "You've got to—"

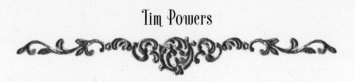

"What do we need two shillings for?" interrupted Harriet.

Skate glared at her. "There's no way you two can swim a mile upriver at this hour, wouldn't you agree? Your only hope is to find a coach—wheels make no footprints, I can tell you that—so *run* now to St. Paul's, you'll be able to find a coach on the Strand. Take it to the horse ferry below Westminster Palace. There's probably a barge moored there, by what used to be Thorney Island in long ago times—you've heard of Nobody's Home?"

Jacky shook her head, but Harriet drew in her breath. "Is he real?" she asked. "And does he really take blood for pay?"

"So I've heard," said Skate. "But I've known people go to him and come back no worse. Those shaders or their kind, on the other hand, will leave you dead."

Jacky glanced up and down the moon-lit street, trying to see if a waving shadow lurked in some recessed doorway. "Who is he?" she asked.

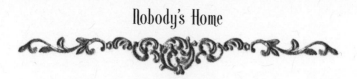

"Nobody, who else?" said Skate impatiently. "The barge is his home. Go!"

Skate wheeled his cart to the wall of St. Swithin's as Jacky and Harriet began running west through the patches of moonlight and darkness, and when Jacky glanced back over her shoulder she saw the legless man swing the spectacles against the London Stone.

"Thimble and pea?" asked Harriet breathlessly when the two of them had waved down a stray hackney coach by the broken statue of Queen Anne in front of the cathedral, paid the driver and told him their destination, and climbed in and pulled the door closed. The leather seats were still warm, and the interior of the coach smelled of very recent perfume and cigar smoke.

Jacky yawned, more from nervousness than because of the late hour, and she flexed

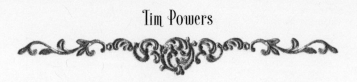

her hands gingerly. "I put a pea under one of three pewter thimbles on a table, and slide them around, and then chaps bet on which thimble the pea is under. But I switch in a hollow pea made of India rubber, and I can hide it flat between my fingers and make it appear, or not, under any thimble. They lose their money. What do you mean, he takes blood for pay?"

She heard the driver flip the reins, and then she was rocked back in her seat as the horses stepped briskly forward and the coach lurched into motion.

"You say your Doggy Joe fellow is real," said Harriet, "not just a frighty tale—maybe Nobody is too. Folks say he lives on a boat, and can shuffle ghosts up or down. I've heard he's a ghost himself, which likely makes it easier."

"But why blood?"

"I don't know," said Harriet, more loudly to be heard over the grinding of the wheels on the pavement, "Ghosts like blood?" She

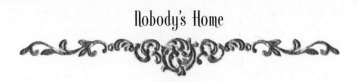

touched her neck. "I'm glad you knocked me down. Even so I've got blisters and I can feel a good deal of my hair's gone."

Neither of them spoke then, and for several minutes they simply huddled in their coats and watched rows of dark buildings shift past like derelict galleons on an outgoing tide.

The Strand widened as the coach rattled past St. Clement Dane's on its island in the middle of the road, and Jacky told herself that she had *not* just seen a cluster of dark, waving figures between the pillars of the western portico. Clouds had again eclipsed the moon, and outlines and relative distances were obscure.

"Why hopscotch?" she asked quickly.

"Well, hopscotch *there*, by the stone," replied Harriet. "In times past, anyway. It's supposed to wake up your ghost, so he's right clinging to you, and then you hop him through the seven squares of Purgatory, saying his name at each square, and then jack

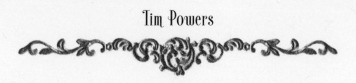

him right out at the top. He's supposed to disappear—not *set you on fire*." She shook her head. "It's a sin, too, unnatural, like you're trying to force God's machinery. You got to do it on one foot, so you're touching the ground some, but not all the way. I wonder if it's still a sin if it doesn't work."

Jacky thought it probably was, but didn't say anything.

They alighted from the coach in front of a pub called the Portman Arms at the corner of Wood and Millbank Streets, a hundred yards down from the ornately Gothic south wall of the Palace of Westminster. The pub's windows were dark, and the warehouses on the east side of the street looked abandoned. Jacky forlornly watched the coach rattle away north, back toward streets with occasional lighted windows, and shivered.

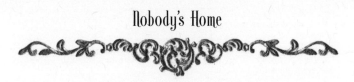
A very dark alley between two of the warehouses led away in the direction of the nearby river, and Harriet waved toward it.

"The horse-ferry is that way," she said, her soft voice barely audible in the cold wind that funneled down the street.

Jacky eyed the dark gap unhappily. "Maybe our ghosts have gone back to sleep again, now that we're so far away. We could wake up the landlord at the Portman, just get a room."

Harriet reached out and touched the glass vial hanging on Jacky's shirt, and then jerked her hand back. She quickly looked up and down the patchily-moonlit street, and she stiffened when she looked north, toward the palace.

"To the river," she whispered, "fast."

Jacky glanced north as she hurried after her companion, and she broke into a sprint when she saw two dark figures up at that end of the street, moving toward them as smoothly as billows of smoke.

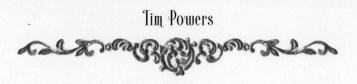

The alley echoed to the fast knocking of the girls' footsteps—ghosts can see footsteps! thought Jacky—and the air between the close brick walls was heady with the scents of tobacco and cinnamon. When they burst out into the moonlight again, between two docks that stretched out over the black water, Jacky was panting and glad of the fresh breeze in spite of its biting chill.

Harriet was looking up and down the dark pebbled shore, her hair whipping around her face. A couple of barges were canted over against scaffolding up on the slope, a set of steel tracks led down the slope and right into the river, a row of stout posts stood up in the shallows—but Jacky couldn't see any particular barge that might be Nobody's Home, and over the wind she could hear flapping and echoing whispers from the alley behind them.

"There!" cried Harriet, pointing north and breaking into a run.

Jacky followed without having seen what her companion might have pointed at, and

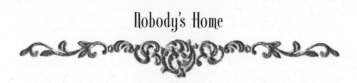
the breath whistled through her teeth as her boots pounded over the clattering wet stones. Her hat flew away, unnoticed. For a moment the two girls were hunched over in fish-reeking darkness as they dodged pilings under one of the docks, and then they were out under the cloudy sky again and a low vessel was visible anchored in the shallows to their right, with dim green light showing at three portholes barely above the water line.

Harriet ran splashing straight out into the water, so Jacky followed, hooting in whispers at the icy chill of the water surging up quickly from her ankles to her thighs. She peered ahead at the vessel—it was a low wooden barge with a smokestack and no masts, perhaps twenty feet long from its blunt bow to its raised stern, and she could now see a ladder amidships that hung down into the water between a couple of the portholes. Canvas-bag fenders hung at the bow and stern.

Harriet had lunged forward and was swimming now, and Jacky gritted her teeth and did

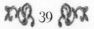

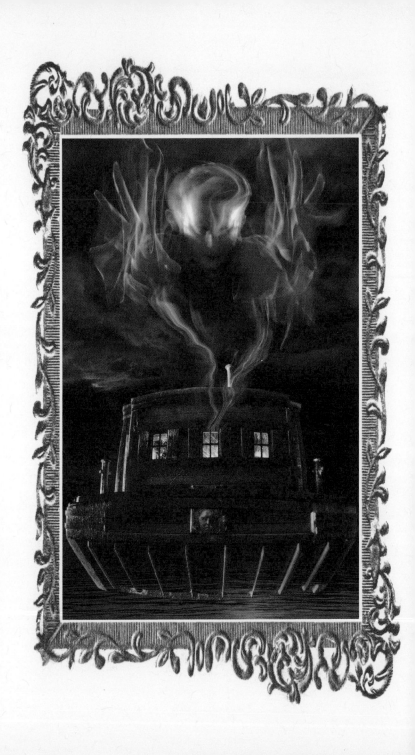

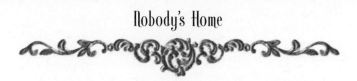
the same, rigidly keeping her head above the rippling water. She craned her neck to look back—two wavering man-like shapes hung where the waves lapped the stones.

At the ladder, the two girls clung to a rung above the water, panting and shivering. "Why are you," gasped Harriet, "*so* desperate to—lose your lover's ghost?"

Jacky just shook her head miserably, freezing in the water but dreading the wet climb up into the cold wind.

"I mean—" Harriet's voice came out in spasmodic rushes, "*he* doesn't want—to burn *you* up—does he?"

"I—don't want to have to—burn *him* up."

Harriet waited another moment, then resolutely climbed up the ladder. Jacky followed, gripping the rungs with numbed hands, and when she pulled herself up to the gunwale she heard Harriet say, "Permission to—come aboard—sir."

Jacky rolled over the gunwale and fell onto the deck and hugged herself in the momentary

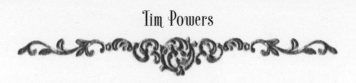

shelter from the wind; the flintlock pistol in her belt dug into her stomach, and it occurred to her that it wasn't going to be useable any time soon. She could see Harriet crouched beside her, and, focusing past her, a short man standing on the deck a few yards away in a slouch hat and a long oilskin coat. In the intermittent moonlight Jacky saw the gleam of spectacles on the man's round face.

The face looked up, toward the shore, and then down again at the two girls on the deck.

"Permission yes," the man said softly.

Below deck the main cabin was in the stern, and the ceiling was high enough for them to stand up straight, and wide enough so that the three occupants weren't crowded together. A big upright boiler in the stern radiated welcome heat from the closed iron door of its firebox, and the smells on the

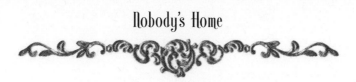

warm air were a peculiar mix of chocolate and the juniper reek of gin; and two lamps with green glass panes shed an underwater glow over everything.

Jacky looked around the cabin nervously. A narrow linen tent was set up against the forward bulkhead, between two low doors; closer to hand, a wooden table was bolted to the deck, and on it, beside three octavo-size leatherbound books, stood a clay jar with Greek letters pressed into its sides and a small hole near the bottom; and railed shelves at every height held an assortment of books and glass jars and mismatched shoes.

Jacky was avoiding looking at their host, and when she glanced down at the puddles she and Harriet were leaving on the deck she noticed a line of seven foot-wide squares and a wide circle painted in white, or possibly pale green, on the polished boards. Hopscotch again. The pattern might have extended farther, for the circle at the far end of the squares was right up against the skirts of the tent.

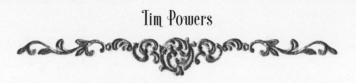

"Oftentimes, more than you suppose," the man said in a quiet uninflected voice as he shrugged out of his oilskin coat and hung it and his hat on a bulkhead hook, "swimming is the way to this. Clothing that's wet should be put in there," he said with a wave toward the low doors forward, "and dry ones put on."

At last Jacky lifted her head and looked at him. He was hardly more than five feet tall, and his nondescript flannel shirt and corduroy trousers didn't look new. The spectacles seemed to make his eyes appear smaller and more distant than they could really have been, and his face was round and smooth under wisps of fine fair hair that looked green in the peculiar lamplight. It occurred to her that it was an entirely unmemorable face—if she were to meet him again she wouldn't be sure it was the same man.

Whenever Jacky shifted her position on the gently rocking deck, she was freshly and uncomfortably aware of her cold, sodden

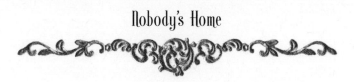

clothing, and "dry ones" sounded wonderful, but she began, "What we want—"

The man held up a pale hand, then nodded toward the clay jar on the table. "A clepsidra there, a water clock. Into it can be put a ghost, so refreshment of the water keeps in your house his spirit. Into those books, as well, if one reads them every month. Or lamps he'll bide in, while the oil goes replenished."

Jacky looked anxiously at the two green lamps mounted at shoulder height on the port and starboard bulkheads, and the man was faintly smiling at her when she looked at him again.

"But it's not for keeping the ghost that you've come, I think. It's expulsion through," he said, glancing at the hopscotch pattern on the floor, "Purgatory. Forever away from here."

Jacky touched the vial that still hung around her neck—and it was as hot as ever. "No, I want to keep mine. I just want him put back the way he was before tonight. Not... waked up and following me."

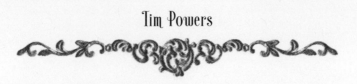

"Was?" said the man.

Jacky stepped closer to the boiler firebox and held her hands out to the radiated heat; the gin-and-chocolate smell was beginning to make her feel sick. "Like in your aspidistra," she said, nodding toward the water clock. "I just want his spirit near me, so I can feel him *with* me still, but doing no more than putting his rhymes into my head when I'm sleepy, like before. Not…*banishing* him. I just want you to cool the ashes of his dottle again."

"That means ashes from a pipe," spoke up Harriet, moving to stand beside Jacky by the firebox, "not his head." Jacky nodded and touched the hot glass vial hanging on her shirt.

"Who is your ghost?" the man asked Jacky. His voice was no louder, but it seemed to echo as if he spoke from some distance down a tunnel.

"His name? Colin Lepovre. He was my fiancee. A poet." He kept staring at her, so she added, "He was murdered by Dog-Face Joe, if you've heard of him?—can switch bodies with

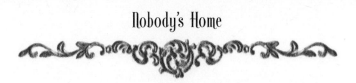
people?—and has to do it a lot because each body he takes for himself starts to grow fur all over it?" The man nodded again, still with no expression, so Jacky went on, forcing her voice to be level. "Dog-Face Joe took Colin's body, and switched Colin into a cast-off body—one with fur all over it and a, a stomach freshly full of poison."

"Were you once in a different body yourself?"

Jacky blinked at him. "What? No. Why— oh hell. The moustache is a fake." She touched it, and found that it was already askew on her upper lip; she pulled it off and shoved it into a pocket. "I'm a girl." Somehow she had thought this magician, or whatever he was, would have known that.

"Ah." He stared into her eyes for several uncomfortable seconds, then looked away. "Pardon—living bodies are not prominent in my vision."

After another pause, Harriet said quietly, "I'm a girl too, just for clearness sake.

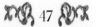

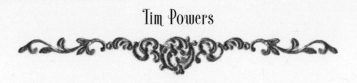

And I want *my* ghost all the *way* gone, like you said."

The man nodded. "Compelling them can be done." He waved in the direction of the shore. "Thorney Island this was once, straddled away from the mainland by branches of the Tyburn, a stream under pavement now. On the island King Canute eight hundred years ago ordered stopping to the tide—that is, the ghosts in the river. The river didn't stop, but the ghosts did. Still they do, here."

Jacky turned around to warm her back and stare at the man. "Are you Nobody?"

"Who else?"

"You take blood, in payment for your services?"

"A drop." He shrugged. "Two drops, maybe three."

Jacky bared her teeth and rolled her eyes— she recalled Harriet saying, *it's a sin, too, like you're trying to force God's machinery*—and finally she stamped on the deck. "If I *don't* do this," she said, her voice catching in her throat,

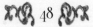

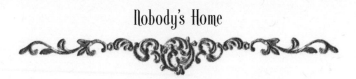
"will he follow me, face me?" She hoped that if tears spilled down her cheek they'd be mistaken for river water. "*Speak* to me?"

Nobody pointed a pudgy finger at the vial on her chest. "Yes. You saw him, I think. Nearby now he waits for you."

Jacky exhaled shakily. "Then I can spare quite a few drops." She stepped away from the boiler toward the doors in the forward bulkhead, and Harriet was right behind her.

Jacky and Harriet each crouched through one of the doors on either side of the narrow linen tent, and in the darkness beyond hers, Jacky felt her way for a couple of feet and soon touched the back bulkhead of what must have been a storage closet. Her boots had tangled in a length of cloth, and when she unsnagged it and felt it, she concluded that it was some sort of heavy woolen nightshirt. After a moment's

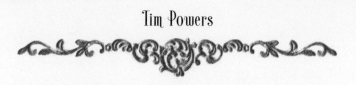

wary hesitation she decided that it would do, and that the possibility of her clothing being stolen here was remote, and so she tugged her wet clothes and boots off and pulled the woolen garment on over her head. She was unarmed, but the Nobody fellow didn't seem strong, and if he tried anything she'd brain him with his clytemnestra or whatever the thing was called.

She pushed open the door and was startled again by the green radiance from the two lamps—*lamps he'll bide in,* she thought, *while the oil goes replenished*—as the other door opened and Harriet came out on her hands and knees, blinking. Jacky saw that they were both now wearing white robes— her own a bit wet and grimy in spots from being stepped on. The deck was chilly under her bare feet.

"The pistol would be good to have," spoke up Nobody, who had pulled a stool out from under the table and was now sitting down. His hands were open and palm-up in front of him.

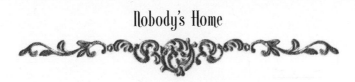
"It's, uh, soaked," Jacky pointed out.

"Good to have," repeated Nobody.

Jacky shrugged, stepped back into the storage locker and returned with her dripping flintlock; after glancing around the cabin, she laid it beside the clay jar on the table.

The man smiled, exposing two rows of little rounded teeth, and the boat shook as if it had run aground. White light flickered for a moment outside the portholes.

He took no visible notice of it. He opened a cabinet on the starboard bulkhead and fetched out an inkpot, a pen, and two sheets of paper, and he laid them on the table beside Jacky's pistol.

"Dip the pen in the ink," he said to Harriet, "and hold it and one of the papers." When she had complied, he asked her, "Who is your ghost?"

She visibly took a deep breath and squared her shoulders. "My husband, Moraji. He was from India. We were married almost three years ago, had two babies who died. He died a

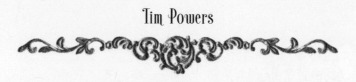

month ago, falling from a roof. Now that he's dead he wants to burn me up."

The man nodded, as if this was not uncommon. He turned again to the cabinet, and this time it was a pint bottle of gin and a bowl of chocolate squares that he set down on the table. For a grotesque moment Jacky thought he was offering them refreshments.

But, "Ghosts will come to candy and liquor," he said, stepping away now toward the tent.

"Moraji didn't like candy," said Harriet unsteadily, "and he didn't drink."

"I said *ghosts*," said Nobody. "Where you stand is up here, by the circle. Both, both."

Jacky and Harriet padded across the deck and stood beside the tent, and Nobody pulled the linen flap to one side; within stood a rough column of stone, four feet high and two feet wide, broken off on top. It looked like impure jade in this light, but when Nobody took off his spectacles and struck them against the stone, Jacky guessed what it was.

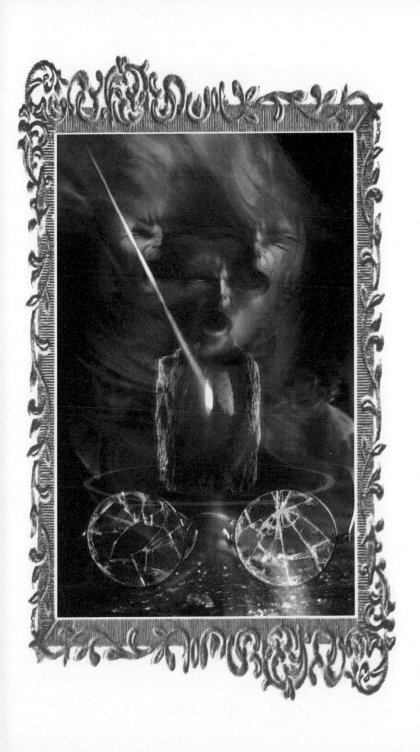

"The other piece of the London Stone," she said.

"We were just there," said Harriet faintly.

Dropping the eyeglasses, both lenses of which were shattered, Nobody turned to the girls; his face was blank, and his eyes still seemed unnaturally small in his round face, like two raisins in a pudding.

The gin bottle rattled on the table, and several of the chocolate squares burst apart.

"Yes," he said, and his voice was now definitely echoing. "The greater piece. A hundred years ago the Worshipful Company of Spectacle Makers used to break eyeglasses like these on it, on holy days, with priests in attendance and green stones in a hopscotch pattern on the street. And I've broken on it the lenses that held your ghosts."

A sudden cold wind was blowing across Jacky's bare ankles, and when she spun around she saw a streak of white moonlight on the ladder that led to the upper deck; the hatch-cover was open, or gone. She wondered

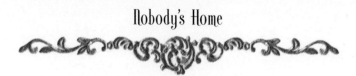
if it might have blown off its hinges until she saw two undissipating smoky columns standing now over there by the ladder; even as she watched, branching wisps coalesced into arms that bent and straightened and bent again, and billows at the tops paled and condensed into angular heads.

She looked away quickly, her heart pounding in her chest. Was one of those awful figures Colin's ghost? Her hand darted to her chest, but the vial on the ribbon wasn't there; she realized that she had left it with her clothes in the storage locker.

Harriet was looking past her toward the ladder, and her face was pale green in the emerald lamplight, her lips sucked tightly over her teeth. Jacky knew her own face must look the same.

"Write his name on the paper," Nobody called to Harriet, "and then go stand on the first square. Both feet, no need of hopping while we're on flowing water." When she hesitated and threw a frightened glance toward

Jacky, he added, "He won't molest you—he will be bound by all he is now, his name."

Harriet bowed her head and scribbled on the paper, using her left hand as a backing— Jacky was relieved to see that she knew how to write—and then, looking only down at the deck, she hurried to stand in the first square.

One of the spidery figures by the ladder waved its jointed arms over its head, and a windy hissing from it contorted into recognizable words: *"You come with me!"*

"Do not speak!" said Nobody quickly to Harriet. "Write the name again, and step into the second square."

The hissing kept up as Harriet slowly made her way through six more squares, spasmodically writing the name again before stepping into each one, but after its first statement the faintly articulated noise sounded only like the twittering of birds.

When Harriet was standing unsteadily in the seventh square, Nobody told her to halt. From a shelf near the cabinet he took a glass

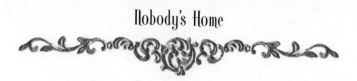

jar and another pen and crossed to where Harriet stood swaying. Peering more closely, Jacky saw that the new pen appeared to be made of bone, and that it was bristly with points at the nib end.

He handed Harriet the pen and with trembling pudgy fingers unscrewed the lid of the jar. "River water," he said. "Dip the pen and write the name once more."

Harriet winced as she gripped the pen, and when she dipped it into the jar Jacky saw blood on the girl's fingers. Harriet gingerly scribbled the name one more time, though the water left no visible track on the paper.

"Crumple the paper," said Nobody hoarsely, "and drop it into the circle below the stone."

Jacky was glancing at Nobody when the ball of paper tapped the deck, and she saw him inhale deeply—and her ears popped and the tent flap twitched; and just for that moment the man's blank face was darker, and sharpened into distinct features, and a deep sigh escaped the now-clearly-drawn mouth; and looking the other way, Jacky saw that only one dark swaying figure stood by the ladder now.

Her gaze swung back to Nobody, and his face had subsided into its previous pallidly unlined anonymity.

The ghost didn't go away to any afterlife, she thought dizzily, it never made it as far as the stone. This Nobody fellow *ate* it. Nobody's prickly bone-pen took Harriet's blood and then through that link he inhaled her husband's ghost.

Jacky yawned, and her ears popped back to normal hearing.

"It's gone," said Nobody, and Harriet sat down abruptly and buried her face in her hands, breathing deeply. Both pens rolled away across the deck.

"Now yours," said Nobody, turning his moon face to Jacky. "To be put back quiescent into that small bottle—" He leaned closer to her, blinking. "Which you have put where?"

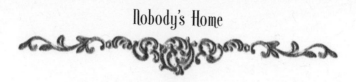

Nobody's Home

The wind over the river must have picked up; a draft had begun whistling somewhere in the cabin.

Jacky's face was cold with sweat. "I left it in that closet. But is he going to *speak* to me?" She pointed at Harriet. "Hers *spoke* to her."

Harriet, still sitting on the floor, looked up at her bleakly. "You're more afraid of yours than I was of mine."

Jacky looked toward the ladder; the wobbling form still stood there, slowly bending its arms and twisting its head. Then she crouched beside Harriet.

"He came to my house," she said to her in a fast whisper, "my parents' house. He was in a stranger's body, covered with fur and dying of poison, and Dog-Face Joe had chewed the tongue to ribbons before he switched Colin into it, but—Colin managed to *come to me*, because—because he loved me." Jacky took a deep, hitching breath. "Damn it, it was midnight and—and I heard the front door bang open, and then what seemed to be a

59

big gorilla with blood all over its mouth came rushing up the hall at me! There was a pistol—" She nodded toward the table, "—that one—and I—how in *Hell* could I have known it was Colin?"

Harriet whispered, "You shot him?"

The windy whistling was louder.

Jacky closed her eyes and nodded. "And when he was dying there on the floor in front of me, I looked into his eyes and—his eyes were the wrong color of course, but—we recognized each other. We both knew I had killed him. And then he died." She balled her fists. "I can't face him, have him *speak* to me!"

"But it was that, that Dog-Face Joe person who really *killed* him."

Jacky shook her head. "I fired the ball that pierced his heart."

The blowing draft had a hollow sound now, not whistling anymore, and then it rose in pitch and formed the word *Jacky*.

Jacky spun, still crouching, and stared at the thing by the ladder.

"…Colin…!"

The wind said, *"Is it you? I can't see."*

"Do not be approaching it," said Nobody. "Fetch your pendant and I will put the ghost back in, and cool it to sleep."

"Yes," said Jacky, looking away from the ghost and getting to her feet, "quickly." He inhaled Harriet's husband's ghost, she thought, but he can't do that with Colin's. I'll be able to sense it if Colin's ghost—sleeping again, merciful God!—is put back in the vial.

She had taken two steps toward the storage locker when the ghost voice said, *"Let me go."*

Jacky turned to the infuriatingly empty face of Nobody. "Is he—it—aware? Of us, what we're saying?"

"As an imbecile would be."

Harriet had stood up too, and now put her hand on Jacky's shoulder. "It's not him," she said. "There's not enough there to really *want* anything."

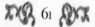

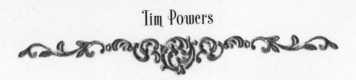

Jacky heard a high, whispered note that might have been a wail. *"Jacky,"* said the voice, *"are you here? I'm alone."*

Even as Nobody opened his small mouth to forbid it, Jacky turned to face the thing across the deck and called, "I'm here, Colin!" Her voice scraped her throat. "And you won't be alone, you'll be with me all the time, just like you were before tonight!"

"Let me go where I am."

The airy voice had no inflection. Jacky blinked tears out of her eyes and peered at the dim figure in the green radiance, trying to see any expression, any face in it.

Go where I am? she thought. Does it want to rejoin Colin's departed soul? She thought of figures in dreams, and wondered if they felt lost when the dreamers awakened and turned their attention to the affairs of the day.

Harriet was peering at the fingers of her own right hand, which had held the wounding pen, and then she looked narrowly at Nobody.

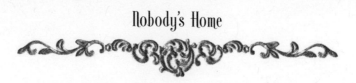
"Don't do the hopscotch," she said to Jacky.

Jacky glanced to the side at her, and momentarily wondered if Harriet guessed that Nobody had cheated her and simply consumed the ghost of her husband.

"If it says—" began Jacky.

"It doesn't *know* what it's saying," Harriet said.

"Its words are like numbers on rolled dice," said Nobody. He did his boneless-looking shrug again. "Fetch the pendant or pick up the pens."

It doesn't matter, Jacky thought, what the ghost may want, even if it is distinct enough to want something; if I do the hopscotch trick, Nobody will inhale Colin's ghost, and I will *not* permit that, I will *not* see Colin's remembered features briefly animate Nobody's stagnant face.

"I'll get the pendant," said Jacky, and she trudged barefoot across the deck to the door in the forward bulkhead and pulled it open.

When she was in the narrow locker and had pulled the door closed behind her, she crouched and felt through her tumbled wet clothing, and she found a fold of cloth that was hot; she flipped the fabric this way and that, and soon disentangled the ribbon with the vial attached to it.

But she had felt something hard in another bundle of wet cloth, and she dug around until her fingers found their way into a pocket and closed on three little cylinders—her thimbles. Probably the India rubber pea was in that pocket too, but she didn't bother to feel for it.

She stood up in the darkness and draped the ribbon around her neck; immediately she could feel the heat of the vial through the cloth of the robe. And after a long moment's thought she closed her fist on the three pewter thimbles.

She opened the door and stepped back into the cabin. Harriet and Nobody were still standing on this side of the hopscotch pattern,

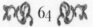

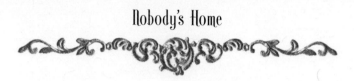
and Colin's ghost bobbed its shadowed head on the far side by the ladder.

"What do I do?" she asked.

The man reached out to the green-glass lamp on the starboard bulkhead and lifted the conical iron cap from the top of it; Jacky winced, for it must have been very hot, but Nobody's face continued to show no expression as he reversed the cap and set it back in place. It was now a concave vessel, and he began picking up the chocolate squares from the bowl and dropping them into the inverted cap. Smoke sprang up immediately, and the coffee-like smell of burned chocolate filled the cabin.

He lifted the bottle of gin, but just held it and extended his other hand toward Jacky.

"Give me the pendant," he said.

"What will you do?"

His little eyes darted to the smoking chocolate and back to her. "Quickly," he said.

"But—what?"

"I will put it into the burning candy, which will draw and hold the ghost, and then

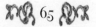

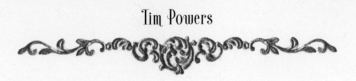

pour the liquor in. It will burn, and his false alertness will burn away with it. Sleep again... is what he will have again, in the little glass jar of yours."

The ghost's windy whisper intruded then, repeating her name.

"Oh please!" she cried to the thing without looking at it, "just be silent for a minute!"

It said her name again.

"Speaking to it is not good," said Nobody.

But Jacky discovered that she had to. "We'll be like we were," she called in a pleading tone, still not looking in that direction, "you—quiet, invisible, but—there." In a blessedly minimal way, she added to herself. "Us together. I—*need* you—like that. *Damn* it," she added, and with her free hand she pulled the ribbon off over her head and thrust it toward Nobody. "Do it fast."

The whistling voice formed words again: *"It spreads its wings, unmindful of the height..."* and Jacky helplessly recalled the second line of the couplet: *And takes the*

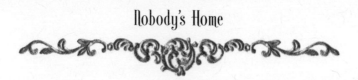
wind in half-forgotten flight. It was the end of one of Colin's sonnets, about a long-confined bird finally set free. Jacky turned a stricken look on the agitated ghost across the cabin.

She caught Nobody's loose-skinned wrist. "I didn't know it was you," she said in a quiet but intense voice, speaking now to the pendant in Nobody's hand. She forced the words out. "God help me, I didn't know I was killing *you.*"

"Forgive," said the thing by the ladder.

Jacky raised her head and made herself look at it. "Do you," she whispered hesitantly, "mean you…forgive me?"

"All," it said.

Jacky found that she took that statement, vague as it was and from a doubtful source, as definitive assent. Tears were running down her cheeks, but her shoulders relaxed and she wondered if they had been tensed ever since Colin's death a month ago.

She released Nobody's wrist.

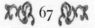

The ghost went on, *"He yearns to be away who cherished thee,"* it said, *"let nothing of his spirit here remain."* Those lines were paraphrased from another of Colin's poems. And then the voice added, *"I forgive, you forgive. Forgive all, release all."*

After two jolting heartbeats Jacky seized Nobody's hand, which had now moved so close to the hot iron cup that she burned her knuckles against its edge.

And she pulled the pendant and ribbon out of Nobody's fist.

"No," she said dully, "I must lose him twice." In her other hand she squeezed the three thimbles, and she said to Nobody, "Let's do the hopscotch."

Jacky wrote *Colin Lepovre* in ink on the other piece of paper.

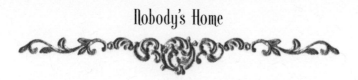
"Drop the vial onto the first square," said Nobody, "and then stand in it."

Seven squares of Purgatory, she thought as she stepped into the square. It was rings, in Dante. *It's a sin, too*, Harriet had said. Was this token Purgatory for Colin's ghost, or for herself?

Six more times she wrote his name and picked up the vial to drop into the next square, and each time she picked it up the vial seemed cooler. At last she stood in the seventh square, with the circle and the London Stone in front of her.

"Halt," said Nobody.

She looked to the side and saw him dipping the bristly bone pen into the jar of river water; and while he was doing that she slipped the pewter thimbles onto her thumb and the first two fingers of her right hand. And when he handed her the dripping pen she kept the tips of her fingers folded in.

Harriet opened her mouth to say something, but Jacky frowned and shook her head at her.

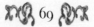

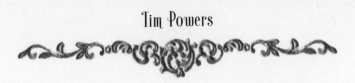

She made sure to wince realistically as she gripped the bristly pen with her shielded fingertips and clumsily wrote Colin's name one last time, in water, unreadably. The bone-spines scratched harmlessly against the thimbles; no blood was drawn.

"Crumple the paper," said Nobody hoarsely, "and drop it and the pendant into the circle below the stone."

This time Jacky didn't look at Nobody; she watched the paper and the glass vial strike the deck, and she saw a thin streak of light that shifted from green to bright white as it sprang from the vial and made a momentary spot of light on the surface of the stone.

She heard the wind of Nobody's inhalation—and it didn't stop. Again her ears popped, and the flap of the linen tent was fluttering in a new breeze.

She spun to look toward the ladder, and the cloudy figure was smaller—a patch of fog, a curl of diaphanous silk, a ripple in moonlight.

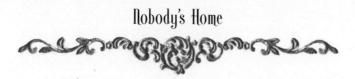
Over the whistiling of Nobody's con-
tinuing inhalation, she heard a tiny voice
whisper, clearly, *"Finish it, my love—act it
out the same—I need it to look the same—you
again, and me again, and the same pistol…"*

She didn't even need to hear the flintlock
pistol rattling on the table to know what it
meant. Finish it, she told herself, finish it for
God's sake.

She stumbled past the inflating figure
of Nobody to the table, shook the thimbles
from her hand and snatched up the pistol.
Blinded with tears, she pointed the barrel
toward the ladder, tugged the hammer back
with her thumb and then pulled the trigger.
The hammer struck the empty flash-pan with
a tiny click.

She heard a sound that might have been a
distant glad cry, and then the barge began to
shake itself to pieces.

The boards of the deck overhead were
splintering and bending downward in the
gale that suddenly seemed to be coming from

all directions, and jars were leaping off the shelves to burst in wild spray, but all sounds were muffled as Jacky caught Harriet's arm and pushed her toward the forward bulkhead, in which the storage locker doors were already open and swinging back and forth. The two girls grabbed up their flapping wet clothing and turned toward the ladder.

The figure of Nobody was a huge balloon now, the face just a scatter of bobbing eyes and nostrils around the wide, sucking hole of a mouth on the top of the expanding sphere, the shirt and trousers just torn rags flapping in the wind around the bulbous limbs. Somehow he was still inhaling, uselessly but powerfully, and everything, even the air, was being pulled into him.

The green lamps went dark as they sprang from their hooks. Jacky tugged Harriet forward, and the two of them scrambled in sudden darkness across the deck, covering their faces with their hands to block flying pieces of wood and ignoring fragments of

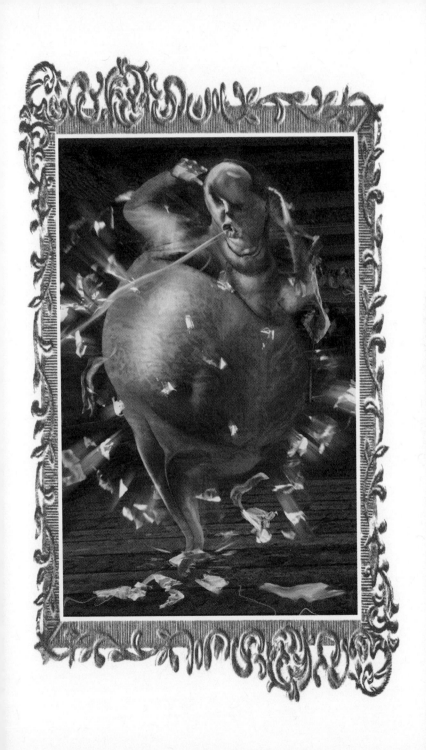

glass cutting their bare feeet, and then they were hurriedly climbing up the flexing ladder.

Out in the moonlight and cold fresh air, they took two running steps across the concave deck and sprang over the gunwale.

The water, when she crashed into it, was colder than Jacky remembered. After she had kicked her way to the churning surface she wasn't able to take a deep breath, and she found it hard to swim while holding the pistol in one hand and what she hoped was most of her clothing in the other, but within a few yards the water was shallow enough for her to wade toward the pebbled shore.

Behind her she heard a loud boom that echoed back from the buildings on the east side of the river, followed by a prolonged tumult of falling water; even as she shifted around against the current to look back, boards were spinning down out of the sky to splash into the river. The wind carried a gust of chilly spray across her face.

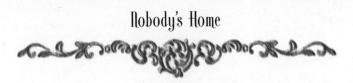

At last she and Harriet were panting on their hands and knees on the wet stones of the shore. Harriet lifted one hand to push her dripping hair away from her face.

"What'd you *do*?" she gasped.

Jacky had laid down her pistol in order to spread her sopping jacket out on the pebbles, though she was shivering so violently that her hands were clumsy. "I—cheated him, I suppose," she managed to say through clenched teeth. Pushing her numbed fingers into the side pocket of the jacket, she fumbled out the soggy false moustache. It looked like a tangle of hair someone might pull from a clogged drain, but she jerkily combed it out with her fingernails and presed it hard against her upper lip.

"It won't—stick," said Harriet.

"It will if I keep my hand on it." Jacky picked up the pistol again. "Men coming."

A square of lamplight shone in the darkness of sheds and docks that made a jagged silhouette against the distant moonlit wall

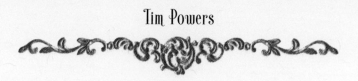

of Westminster Palace, and from moment to moment the yellow light was interrupted by figures running toward the shore. The thudding of their boots grew louder.

"Here's two survivors!" came a nearby call, and then a man in a heavy coat was crouching by them as boots in the darkness crunched closer.

"Are there others?" the man gasped. "We can get boats out."

"Nobody but us," said Jacky, speaking in her deeper voice.

"Nobody? Where is he?"

"He'd be dead," said Harriet. She was sitting on the pebbles, trembling and hugging herself. "We're all that's left."

"I think he—exploded," added Jacky.

"Ah! I follow you. That's good then. Are you injured?"

Jacky thought of their cut feet, but said, "No. Just freezing to death."

"Right, we'll get you into blankets in the watermen's shed. Here, you fellows, give

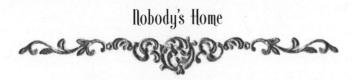

these two a hand. I believe they've rid the river of Nobody."

Huddled in a rough blanket that smelled of old dock pilings but was blessedly dry, and sipping brandy from a tin cup, Jacky kept the knuckle of her free hand pressed against the false moustache. She had explained to their rescuers that her nose would bleed if she let off the pressure.

Two men in worn woollen pea coats and canvas trousers leaned forward from a bench against the wall, their hard faces lit in amber chiaroscuro by the glow from the open door of a coal stove. Smoke curled from a blackened clay pipe clenched between the teeth of one of them.

"But what blew him up?" he asked, speaking around the clay stem, after Jacky and Harriet had described their time on Nobody's Home.

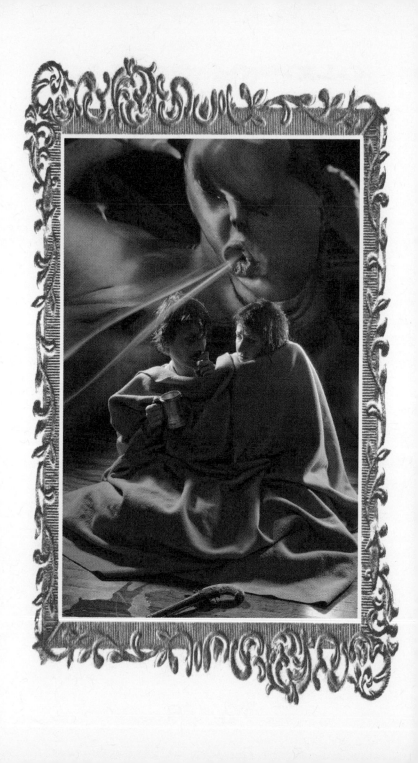

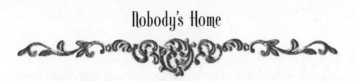

"He cheated me," said Harriet, who was crouched in another blanket beside Jacky. "He used my blood to *eat* my husband's ghost, instead of sending it on to the hereafter. Inhaled the ghost, is what it was. But when it was Jacky-boy's turn, he somehow avoided getting cut by the needles on the pen, and so Nobody didn't get the ghost of...Jacky's brother." Jacky was pleased that her companion was going along with her pretense and her version of the story. "He inhaled, though," Harriet went on, "and when he didn't catch the ghost, it seemed like he couldn't stop inhaling. He blew up like a balloon, and then I suppose he just—popped."

The other man sat back and nodded with evident satisfaction. "It might be years, decades, before he collects again." To Jacky and Harriet he explained, "Ghosts from upriver get snagged here, God knows why, like leaves caught by a drain, and when a whole lot of 'em clump up, they make a sort of man, something very like a man, good enough to talk and naturally good at handling ghosts. It's never what you'd call a particular person—it's Nobody, in that way. And it lives on the smell of fresh blood, like they say jungle plants live on just smells in the air."

"Jungle air, it's got to be," put in his companion. "Damp."

The other man frowned at the interruption. "It wasn't smart for you two to go and try to do business with him. Maybe you know what the priests would say about it. But," he added, shrugging, "it worked out tolerably well. The River Police never really believed the story, and that barge was sometimes there and sometimes not, like some kind of black rainbow that only shows up in moonlight."

The two rivermen got to their feet, and the one with the pipe laid it down on the windowsill. "Dawn soon," he said. "We've got to get the boats out for custom at the stairs. You two can stay here till your things dry out."

"God bless you for rescuing us," said Harriet.

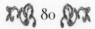

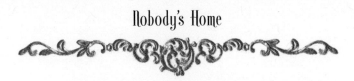

The other man laughed shortly. "You probably saved some *further* idiots that would else have gone aboard that graveyard barge." His companion nodded solemnly.

When they had opened the door to the chilly pre-dawn wind and then closed it behind them, Harriet looked at Jacky.

"Nobody was a ghost himelf," she said. "A compost of a bunch of them, that is. I don't think it was a sin to blow him up."

Jacky gave a brief, mirthless laugh. "Right. What did I do? I killed Nobody."

Harriet nodded uncertainly. "You can toss the moustache now. You've got a mum and da back home? I expect you'll be going back there."

Jacky lifted her hand hesitantly away from her upper lip, and then let her hand fall into her lap when the moustache stayed in place.

"It's sticking again," she said, "now that it's dried out a bit."

"But you can be a girl again now. No need for," Harriet waved toward the pistol that lay on the wooden floor beside Jacky, "*that*, nor the moustache—no need anymore for you to be going into the hell-holes and rookeries."

Jacky frowned at her in puzzlement. "It was Nobody that got killed, not Dog-Face Joe. Nothing about that changed tonight."

The brandy bottle stood on a shelf by the door, and Harriet got up to refill her cup, and then refilled Jacky's too. "We'll have to buy these watermen a new bottle," she said. And when she had sat down beside Jacky and tucked up her blanket, she went on, "You freed yourself from your ghost. He's not there to haunt you anymore."

Jacky swallowed half of the brandy in her cup and closed her eyes as it spread a replacing sort of warmth through her chest. "Was he ever there? Now I think he was never in that flacon of ashes. I believe I only ever imagined his…presence."

Harriet was clearly upset; and as if she were trying to talk Jacky out of another sort of sin, she went on, "He used to recite his poems to you, when you were half asleep!"

"When I was dreaming."

"But you remember—"

"What I remember about this grotesque night I'm sure I'll soon forget. I think the River Police had the story right. What barge? What ghost man?"

"Your—your feet are cut, from broken glass. Mine too."

Jacky nodded. "We were fools to go walking barefoot on the shore at night."

The wind shivered around the watermen's shed.

"Ah." Harriet frowned at Jacky for several seconds, then said, "It was the forgiveness."

Jacky turned to her and said, furiously, "You and I were the only people aboard that barge, if there was a barge at all. What, did I forgive you for something?"

"Your Colin said, 'Forgive…forgive all.' You were glad when it meant he forgave you. For shooting him."

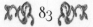

"Colin's been dead for a month. I doubt he has a lot to say now. A ghost's not the person it's a ghost of, you said it yourself."

"If he had stopped with only the one word, when it sounded like he was forgiving you, you wouldn't be doubting all this."

"I don't—"

"He meant for you to forgive the thing that truly killed him, this Dog-Face Joe. He was asking you to give up your revenge."

Jacky clenched her fists. "What if he was? He's gone, taken away from me—if he wasn't gone before tonight, he certainly is now—and I can't…live, I can't resume my life—until that creature that killed him is dead. It's all I have, for now." She exhaled and shook her head. "He's still out there, somewhere."

"But—but you could go home!"

"Until I do this I don't have a home." She held her right hand out in front of her and flexed her fingers. "I feel like I killed myself, too, when I killed Colin a month ago. I'm the

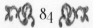

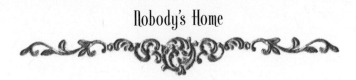
ghost of the girl he was engaged to. Until I do this…I'm nobody myself." She gave Harriet a strained smile and touched her hand. "I'm sorry. In other circumstances I think you and I could have been friends."

Harriet nodded. "I can't argue with you—talk you away from this course."

"No," Jacky agreed. Her shoulders were tense, and she stretched, blinking at the window. "The sun's up, I think. Our clothes and boots should be dry enough to walk away in soon."

Harriet sighed and got up again to refill their tin cups. She paused at the window and looked out at the river, and Jacky could imagine what she was seeing—the early traffic on the river, clouds still edged with coral, the highest wheeling seagulls flashing white in the dawn sunlight.

Jacky's gaze fell to the flintlock pistol on the floor. And she reminded herself that she would have to clean it and oil it soon, so that it wouldn't rust.

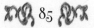

"He is not here; but far away
The noise of life begins again,
And ghastly through the drizzling rain
On the bald street breaks the blank day."

—Tennyson, *In Memoriam*

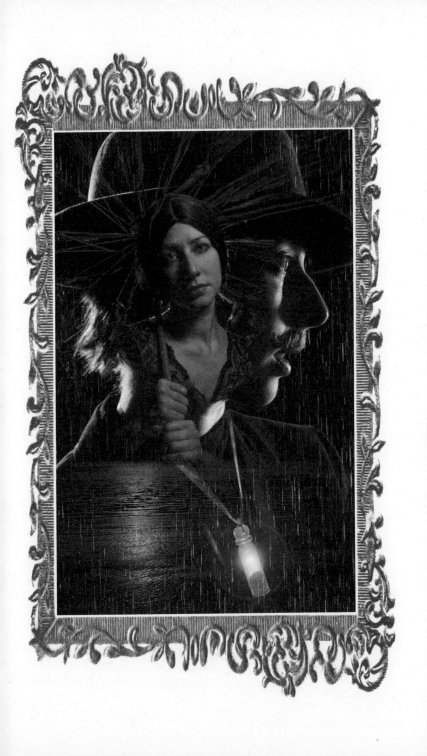